DIETS TO HEL[P]

Colitis, or inflamation of the bow
and this book shows how, wi
programme, the condition can be alleviated naturally.

DIETS TO HELP

COLITIS

by

JOAN LAY
N.D., M.B.N.O.A.

THORSONS PUBLISHING GROUP

First published 1980
First published in this new format 1988`

Lay, Joan
[Diets to help colitis] Diets to help colitis.
1. Man. Colon. Colitis. Therapy. Diet
I. [Diets to help colitis]   II. Title
616.3'4470653   ISBN 0-7225-1704-1

*Published by Thorsons Publishers Limited,
Wellingborough, Northamptonshire, NN8 2RQ, England.*

Printed in Great Britain by B L & U Printing Limited,
Wellingborough, Northamptonshire.

1   3   5   7   9   10   8   6   4   2

CONTENTS

INTRODUCTION

The word 'colitis' tends to be used rather inaccurately to include anything from a prolonged bout of simple diarrhoea – through mucous colitis to ulcerative colitis. The actual meaning is: 'inflammation of the colon'. The colon is the large intestine at the end of the digestive tract, where some absorption occurs, and the waste matter is moved on by muscular contractions at regular intervals.

Colitis is characterized, in its simplest form, by frequent watery stools of a forceful nature accompanied by low abdominal discomfort or pain commonly known as 'colic'. This stage is usually followed by a period of constipation until the colon is sufficiently irritated again to produce a violent effort once more to expel the waste matter in diarrhoea. The vicious circle continues in this way if nothing is done, or if suppressive measures are taken to stop the diarrhoea, until the body, in its effort to get rid of the continued pollution, uses even more drastic methods. The irritated mucous lining of the colon secretes excessively and is expelled with the stools in thready strings. This can continue for some time before the excessive activity of the mucous membrane actually causes the wall of the colon to become thinner. Then breakdown can occur and ulcerations form in small areas, and blood and pus can be seen in the stools.

The standard treatments are all aimed at relieving symptoms, which temporarily make the patient more comfortable, but do not get at basic causes. Drugs and diets are recommended to stop the diarrhoea thus preventing elimination, however faulty, of toxic matter. Nothing is done to improve the state of the colon, and once the bout has been stopped, the whole cycle repeats itself. Sometimes the patient is also tranquillized to avert the worry syndrome, but this does not help in combating it, and merely reduces the quality of life.

The only satisfactory way of treating disease is in taking the person as an entire being, not divided up into compartments and labelled by symptoms. The patient can only be made healthy again by healthy or whole measures, using whole unprocessed foods, fresh air (when it can be found), water, exercise and right thinking. These very simple things can be assisted by vitamin, mineral and herbal supplements in the short run, but in the long run the way of living needs to be reviewed.

CHAPTER ONE

CAUSES OF COLITIS

The causes are numerous and varied, and each sufferer has his own unique pattern. Throughout all cases, however, there are certain factors that persistently appear, and these could be regarded as basic causes.

Digestion

Digestion begins in the mouth with the breaking-up of foods into small particles by thorough chewing and then the mixing of these particles with saliva. This facilitates swallowing and preparing the food to be worked on by the ferments in the stomach. Starch foods actually begin being worked on in the mouth by enzymes in the ptyalin of the saliva. This first step is essential for good digestion, but it is interesting to note how many of the ordinary foodstuffs today are soft and bulkless. White bread can be chewed a little but before it is *thoroughly* broken up and mixed with the saliva it slides into the stomach incompletely prepared. The same thing occurs with puddings and cakes; even most cereals though crisp at first dissolve into a pappy mass when in contact with fluid and slide into the gullet all too easily. Overcooked vegetables and 'mash' are incompletely prepared and therefore the stomach enzymes cannot properly work on any of these foods. Digestion is slowed down, and fermentation occurs. The unconverted foodstuffs produce gas and this in turn causes distention, discomfort and 'heartburn' all lumped together under the umbrella of 'indigestion'.

All the foregoing phenomena result in nutritional loss because absorption is impaired and energy lost through more having to be expended on the effort to digest, so less is available to the muscles and brain producing the tiredness and lack of concentration so often experienced with 'indigestion'. Then in their turn the intestines and colon suffer because the mineral and vitamin content of the food has been destroyed or not taken up owing to the gas and fermentation; and the lack of fibre and bulk in the food diminishes the stimulation to the gut and constipation ensues – setting up the vicious circle already mentioned.

Nervous and Emotional Stress
Stress causes blocking or inhibition of the sympathetic nerve plexuses, while exciting excessive secretion of adrenalin. This, in turn, upsets the rhythm and function of the digestive tract, so that all the processes of digestion, absorption and excretion become unbalanced.

It can be appreciated, then, how very important it is for sufferers to learn how to avoid stress and emotional turmoil, by relaxing, and thereby releasing the tensions. In addition, it is necessary to be *really* honest with oneself in trying to find out why one reacts with resentment, anger, or fear, and come to understand that a change of attitude is essential in helping the body to resume its normal balance. Revealing phrases often occur during consultation which show those reactions of resentment and fear. For example: 'I work my guts out for them.' or 'They would have the very stuffing out of you.'

It is not surprising that the sufferer centres his attention on the condition often counting the number of visits to the loo, and dwelling on the symptoms. Common reactions are fear of eating anything rough, or with pips, or 'acid'. Indeed, one is encouraged by orthodox advice, to keep to soft foods which tend to be devoid of any healing or nutritional properties. Body weight obviously goes down, and this only adds to the worry and fear. Certainly guidance is needed, and a qualified naturopath should be consulted.

Impoverished Refined Unbalanced Diet
There is a great deal of information available about diets of every sort, and, happily, the wholefood idea is spreading rapidly. Incorrect information and lack of understanding are also common, so a resumé here will be helpful.

The body cells have an inherent blueprint – or intelligence, to work to their optimum good, given the basic material to draw from. Therefore it follows that in illness something is amiss, the various body cells are not getting the necessary materials and become unbalanced or 'ill'.

Convenience foods, tinned, processed dyed and flavoured foods are all unnatural, and not only rob the body of essential minerals, but add a burden of complicated chemicals, some of which may be positively harmful. It is really important to use simple foods, raw fruit and salads, whole grains, beans and pulses; nuts and natural dairy products. Those who eat meat should try to obtain free range poultry, and meat from animals unpolluted by growth hormones and concentrated feed. Some food and drink have a particularly depleting and irritating effect on the digestive tract as a whole. Such things as: coffee and tea; chocolate and sugar; spices and pickles and condiments; alcohol and nicotine (from smoking); also mucous-forming foods like milk, cheese and refined white flour products (bread, biscuits, cakes etc.).

It stands to reason that if the diet is not balanced, the body will suffer. Indeed the whole body will be under par, and coupled with the stress factor already mentioned, and the emotional state of the patient in question, the imbalance will result in diarrhoea, then constipation and, eventually, colitis.

Regular Use of Strong Laxatives
This inevitably follows on from the above. The lack of fibre in the diet, which acts as a natural stimulant to the lining of the colon, and encourages the reflex defecation, results in a sluggish bowel. Particularly so because the whole digestive tract is depleted, missing the good whole unrefined foods necessary for good health. Therefore the automatic urge to defecate is missing (or very weak and so ignored) the waste matter will remain in the lower bowel unexpelled and this can persist for several days until, suddenly realizing the lack of elimination, the patient resorts to a laxative of some sort. Most of these are harsh, causing a 'scouring' effect on the bowel and therefore an extreme reaction in the mucous lining of the tract, which can be so severe that diarrhoea persists for a few days. This is followed by exhaustion in the area after so much activity, constipation recurs, and the whole cycle is set up again.

Prescribed drugs
Some of these, particularly the antibiotics and
sulphonamides, inhibit the natural action of the
intestinal flora and even destroy these beneficial
bacteria. Their action in the normal way is to ingest the
poisonous wastes in the faecal mass and render them
harmless, so if they are destroyed the colon becomes
unhealthy and a state of autotoxaemia is produced.
Nature's method of trying to eliminate these wastes is
increased secretion of mucous in the area. There is also a
fall in the prothrombin content of the blood and a
nicotinic acid deficiency. As a result the vessel walls are
weakened and there is an increased risk of bleeding.
Therefore a colitis can be a side-effect, of drugs
prescribed for some other condition.

Allergy
The most common foodstuffs that react on the digestive
tract to cause symptoms of diarrhoea and flatulence are
milk, fats and gluten. The latter, a nitrogenous part of
the starch of wheat, oats, barley and rye, causes a
condition known as 'coeliac illness' or 'malabsorption
syndrome'. This is, however, a subject on its own;
though it could be mistaken for colitis.

CHAPTER TWO

OUTLINE OF THE DIET

Preparation – Rest and Positive Thinking
Rest is important at the beginning of any radical change
in regime, so that the body's energies can be
concentrated in its effort to normalize and heal. In the
case of colitis, where great fatigue and dehydration
occur, this is essential. The change of diet will be utilized
more fully, and any adverse reactions to it lessened after
a period of rest and relaxation. To start with, two days in
bed, followed by five easy days will provide a break in the
usual routine and relief from the usual daily pressures.
This will provide a firm basis for recovery.

It would obviously be a waste of time to try this new
way of living if one is plagued by doubts and fears about
the outcome. One needs to be as positive as possible,
accepting the fact that there are bound to be variations in
progress.

Calmness and confidence are all-important,
remembering that over-stimulation of the system by
excitement or worry causes an immediate reaction from
the colon and brings on the symptoms.

Breathing
Once the decision is made to follow this method, the first

thing to learn is how to breathe properly. Though this is not a dietetic factor – no diet, however balanced, can be fully effective if breathing is shallow, because the blood stream will not be properly oxygenated and so all functions will be less efficient. In addition, it is through deep slow breathing that relaxation is learnt; and as was stated at the beginning, this is an essential part of the treatment to relieve the emotional stress and tension. A third point, to emphasize the benefit obtained from using the diaphragm properly, is that its mechanical movement in rising and falling exerts slight pressure on the gut, and works as a sort of internal massage. This is valuable in restoring tone and rhythm to the large intestine.

How is it done? Lie comfortably on the back with a small pillow beneath the head and a larger one beneath the thighs for support. Place both hands lightly on the abdomen over the navel. 'Think' the breathing into this area – then gently and slowly inhale and feel the abdomen swelling up under the hands; exhale, and the abdomen sinks down. At first, the ribs may expand as usual and the chest heave up, while the abdomen flattens – the old breathing pattern in fact. To overcome this, voluntarily push the abdominal muscles up when inhaling, and let them go on exhaling and gradually the different feeling will be experienced. A good time to practise is on waking and just before going to sleep. Six breaths is all that is needed and then forget the special technique until the specified time. Remember not to get too involved and worry about it or the good result will be defeated. Regular practice is the thing and the new rhythm will gradually take over – and if there is an occasion to cause anxiety – then a few diaphragmatic

breaths will ease the 'butterflies', and in time, deep
breathing can and will prevent these feelings.

Necessary Nutrients
What particularly do those with colitis need? The
impoverished gut cannot at once cope with the roughage
of raw foods, and to attempt to eat them would cause a
very violent reaction. Slow re-education is the best way.
The body really needs a vitamin and mineral rich source
of nourishment to begin to redress the imbalance and
encourage the arousal of the inherent healing power of
the body. To do this without the roughage, at first means
using vegetable and fruit juices, progressing to gentle
bulk such as that in ripe bananas, brown rice and
blended or liquidized fruit and vegetables.

The whole digestive tract may be so sensitive that
cooked fruit and vegetables may have to be used initially;
for example, steamed carrots and beetroots, baked and
stewed apples and so on. The pectin of apples is very
beneficial.

It cannot be emphasized too much that all the refined,
irritating and harmful foods and drinks must be deleted
and recognized as being not only useless but a definite
hindrance to good health. They should not feature again
in the diet, even after the condition has been cured.

The curative regime needs to be rich in all the B
vitamins to nourish the nervous system; in vitam C to
improve absorption of iron and the health of the blood
vessels; in vitamin P to improve the healthy function of
the mucous membranes. The minerals particularly
needed are iron, magnesium, potassium and zinc. To
provide these essentials, foods rich in vitamin B are:
soya, brown rice, yeast extracts, hazel and peanuts,

millet, lentils, whole grains, liver, sesame seeds. Vitamin C is to be found in citrus fruits, peppers, blackcurrants, parsley, raw vegetables, salads and fruits, sprouted seeds; vitamin P in the cells and pith of citrus fruits – so it is important to eat the flesh of the fruit as soon as one is acclimatized to take it. The minerals can be provided by molasses, grapes and raisins, green leafy vegetables, dried fruits and sunflower seeds. The list could be made longer, but these are some of the important sources. In addition natural, 'live' yogurt will be necessary to re-establish the intestinal flora, and garlic to act as a mucus solvent and antiseptic.

Balanced Meals
It is also advisable not to have too many mixtures of foods at one meal because at best, something is imperfectly digested, tending to produce gases and therefore distension and discomfort. It is better not to mix starches and fruits or starches and animal proteins – the acids in both fruit and meat work on the starches causing fermentation and therefore gases, distension, 'rumblings' and discomfort.

The best combinations are: fresh and dried fruits; nuts; milk; salads with starch (bread or potatoes) or salads with protein (egg, cheese, nuts); animal protein with green vegetables; vegetable protein with green vegetables.

When the digestive tract is very upset, as in this condition, it is better to have only one course – as much as is needed – without following it with a 'sweet'.

Many people with colitis are very concerned about weight loss, and the cleansing period of two to four weeks on a very restricted intake is the chief block in adopting a

Nature Cure regime. It must be understood that however much one 'feeds up' while the colon is inflamed and generally unhealthy, proper absorption cannot take place. Whereas a properly supervised light diet can and does produce, after a time, the gain in weight they so much desire.

Supervision
This booklet will be read by some who are trying to 'go it alone' but it is far better, both because of the stress factor and for more lasting results, to have the advice and support of a qualified naturopath.

Ideally, a few days on water only, then on juices only, would be the way to begin the recuperative process; but this should not be tried unless there is the supervision mentioned above. The plan detailed later will be just as effective, but will take longer in producing tangible results. In either case the patient should think in terms of months rather than weeks. After all, the condition is the result of prolonged faulty living, and re-education is not a quick process.

Notes for Following the Cleansing Programme

1. Tap-water is heavily chlorinated and boiling removes this. In areas where sodium fluoride has been added to the main supply, bottled water would be better. There are several types available in supermarkets and wine shops – some still and some sparkling – either will do, providing it is natural spring water. The use of boiled or bottled water simply removes possible irritants and when full recovery is made need not be

continued unless there is a preference to do so.

2. Too much salt is irritating and hardening but, as much of the body's salts are lost through the frequent stools, a very little, say a quarter of teaspoonful, may be added to the water when boiling rice. To make it more appetizing a little finely chopped fresh mint can be added, or parsley which is rich in vitamin C.

3. To make carrot juice without an extractor spread a sheet of gauze over a soup plate. Use the fine side of the grater and grate two medium carrots (having scrubbed them) into this cloth – gather it up by the edges so that the carrot pulp is in a bag – then gently twist and squeeze out all the juice. Pour this into a glass and drink at once, though slowly, before the vitamins and minerals become oxidized.

4. Always eat and drink slowly, savouring the food, chew very well and think about the source of the food – how it has developed from earth, water, sun, and has concentrated these elements to feed your body.

5. Food should not be eaten very hot, as it overstimulates.

6. Two or three deep breaths before eating releases tension in the solar plexus (the area in the midriff where one feels 'butterflies' if anxious).

7. When following the day to day plan, only progress if there has been no marked reaction. If there is a temporary increase in diarrhoea keep the same diet for another day until it subsides.

CHAPTER THREE

CLEANSING AND HEALING PROGRAMME

Resting in bed.
1st Day

7 a.m.	Half-tumbler of cooled boiled water or bottled water, sipped slowly
8 a.m.	2 level tablespoonsful of boiled brown rice with 1 level tablespoonful of stewed apple with honey
10 a.m.	Boiled or bottled water as before
12 noon	Brown rice and apple as at 8 a.m.
2 p.m.	Juice from two carrots
4 p.m.	Brown rice and apple
6 p.m.	Boiled or bottled water
8 p.m.	Slippery elm food
10 p.m.	Water plus pure red grape juice (2 fl. oz. or 50ml of each)

2nd Day
Repeat

3rd Day
Repeat, but at 10 a.m. have juice from 2 carrots instead

4th Day
One may, at this stage, be out of bed but taking it easy.
Repeat the same diet

5th Day

7 a.m.	Water
8 a.m.	One ripe banana (or soaked dried banana); 1 tablespoonful of brown rice
10 a.m.	Carrot juice
12 noon	2 tablespoonsful of brown rice with ½ teaspoonful of yeast extract such as 'Vecon' or 'Barmene' plus 1 level tablespoonful of finely grated raw carrot
2 p.m	Juice of 1 sweet apple
4 p.m.	1 banana with rice
6 p.m.	Herb tea – camomile
8 p.m.	Slippery elm food
10 p.m.	Grape juice with 1 tablespoonful of water only

6th Day
Repeat

7th Day
Same, but take neat grape juice at 10 p.m.

8th Day

7 a.m.	Water
8 a.m.	2 tablespoonsful of stewed apple with 1 level tablespoonful of ground almonds
10 a.m.	Carrot juice
12 noon	3 tablespoonsful of brown rice with yeast extract, 2 tablespoonsful of carrot finely grated, plus ½ tablespoonful of finely chopped parsley
2 p.m.	Apple juice
4 p.m.	2 soaked dried bananas
6 p.m.	Camomile tea
8 p.m.	Slippery elm food
10 p.m.	Grape juice

9th Day
Repeat

10th Day
7 a.m.   Apple juice
8 a.m.   Grated raw apple with 1 tablespoonful ground almonds
10 a.m.   Carrot juice
12 noon   3 tablespoonsful of brown rice with yeast extract, 2 tablespoonsful of grated carrot, $\frac{1}{2}$ tablespoonful chopped parsley, 1 teaspoonful of sunflower seeds
2 p.m.   Half an orange to be eaten segment by segment
4 p.m.   2 soaked dried bananas plus 1 tablespoonful of ground almonds
6 p.m.   Camomile tea
8 p.m.   Baked apple with honey, slippery elm food
10 p.m.   Grape juice

11th Day
7 a.m.   Apple juice
8 a.m.   Fresh banana and ground almonds
10 a.m.   Carrot juice
12 noon   Small salad of: grated carrot, grated apple, chopped parsley, sunflower seeds, scalded and skinned tomato and 1 tablespoonful of cottage cheese
2 p.m.   Eat half orange or grapefruit
4 p.m.   2-3 steamed carrots (according to size) with 1 tablespoonful of cottage cheese
6 p.m.   China tea or camomile
8 p.m.   Baked apple and honey, slippery elm food
10 p.m.   Grape juice

12th Day
Repeat

13th Day
7 a.m.   Apple juice
8 a.m.   Grated apple plus 2 tablespoonsful of natural yogurt (honey if needed)
10 a.m.   Carrot juice
12 noon   Small salad as before, but add 2-3 lettuce leaves
2 p.m.   Half orange or grapefruit
4 p.m.   2 steamed potatoes in their skins (remove skin before eating) plus 2 tablespoonsful of steamed cabbage and 2 tablespoonsful of cottage cheese
6 p.m.   China or camomile tea
8 p.m.   1 baked apple and slippery elm food
10 p.m.   grape juice

14th Day
Repeat

End of strict cleansing and healing programme. At this stage the patient may be tempted to give up; either because improvement makes him feel secure and it has all been easy, or because problems have arisen and the setbacks due to the changed habits depress him, and make him feel that nothing will help.

It would be a great mistake to discontinue now – improvement must be maintained in order to re-educate the entire digestive tract thoroughly. Years have been spent in producing the condition, therefore months will be necessary to remove it. It would be wrong to regard the regime as a 'cure'; it should be appreciated as a new way of living, and that by this revision much will be prevented from going wrong in future. Indeed, a new dimension will be added to life by a realization of well-being and harmony because the body is reacting to the balance and wholeness of the diet and functioning at a higher level. Gradually, greater energy will be found; greater ability to cope with problems because the whole attitude has changed to being positive and constructive.

CHAPTER FOUR

THIRD AND FOURTH WEEK DIET

After the strict regime some improvement will be noticed, but it is advisable to proceed slowly. The third week can be spent in altering the pattern by resuming three meals a day with drinks in between, remembering that one may drink half an hour before a meal but not less than two hours after a meal.

It would be helpful to increase the rather limited salad to include lettuce, cress and some finely chopped or sliced red and/or green pepper – these are very rich in vitamin C. One slice of a hundred per cent wholewheat bread can be taken with this meal with a good margarine or unsalted butter. This will provide some of the B vitamins.

It would be as well only to alter one meal at a time, or the stimulus to the digestive tract would be too great at this stage; so the whole week should centre on expanding the lunch little by little, and keeping two days the same before adding something new. If flatulence or diarrhoea occurs, lessen the amount of the new foodstuff until it is tolerated; should there still be a reaction, delete that food, and it can be used later when the tract has become less sensitive. Remember to keep a high resolve, and not to get depressed or thrown off course when such a reaction occurs.

Presuming that all has gone to plan in the third week, the fourth week should be used to develop the evening meal. Millet and soya savouries can be tried. Pasta dishes (brown of course) and lentil savouries. Examples of these are given later in the recipe pages. In addition, the green vegetable content of the meal should be varied and more adventurous, omitting those that are known to cause flatulence: onions, cauliflower, peas, parsnips and turnips. Overcooked brussel sprouts will also be most indigestible. Indeed, it is interesting to note that any *overcooked* vegetable, especially the green variety, can even cause flatulence in those without a digestive problem.

Lightly cooked liver may be included if liked, as it is easily broken down and is a rich source of iron and B vitamins. Chicken (if free-range and unpolluted by hormones) and fish (cod, haddock, plaice; but *not* the rich ones – halibut, salmon, trout, mackerel – or the so-called 'smoked' ones) can be served once a week also if the patient is non-vegetarian. However, the writer will continue on vegetarian diet reform lines. It is of course understood that frying is absolutely out of the question as a method of cooking anything.

The following menus are intended only as a guide. It may be found preferable to remain on the same one for three, even four days; but the ones given do provide an idea of how the dietetic progression should be made.

Maintenance Menus

Menu 1 (days 1 and 2)

First thing:	4 oz. (100g) apple juice
Breakfast:	1 grated raw apple (including skin and core) 1 tablespoonful of soaked raisins 1 tablespoonful of natural yogurt
Mid-morning:	4 oz. (100g) of carrots, juiced
Lunch:	Salad with small amounts of: lettuce, skinned tomato, grated carrot, sunflower seeds (heaped teaspoonful), grated raw beetroot, 2 oz. (50g) cottage cheese
Mid-afternoon:	China tea or herb tea
Evening meal:	1 or 2 steamed potatoes and carrots according to size 1-2 tablespoonsful of steamed and chopped cabbage with poached egg
Bedtime:	4 oz. (100g) red grape juice warmed or cold

The patient should eat enough to satisfy, but not to feel full up. Main course only, without a sweet, will be the pattern for some time yet.

N.B. Each menu to be repeated the following day.

Menu 2 (days 3 and 4)

First thing:	Half tumbler hot water with teaspoonful of honey and slice of lemon
Breakfast:	2-3 soaked dried bananas, 2 tablespoonsful of natural yogurt

Mid-morning:	4 oz. (100g) of carrots, juiced
Lunch:	Salad with small amounts of: lettuce, cress, pepper, grated carrot, sunflower seeds, skinned tomato, 2 oz. (50g) of ground almonds, 1 slice of whole-wheat bread and butter
Mid-afternoon:	China tea, herb tea or apple or grape juice
Evening meal:	Savoury millet, 1 or 2 carrots, 1 or 2 tablespoonsful of green vegetable
Bedtime:	Red grape juice or 'Vecon'

Menu 3 (days 5 and 6)

First thing:	Half tumbler hot water with juice of ½ lemon plus 1 teaspoonful of honey
Breakfast:	Soya or barley flake 'porridge' with soaked raisins and dried skimmed milk
Mid-morning:	'Vecon' or carrot juice
Lunch:	Salad with small amounts of: lettuce, cress, skinned tomato, pepper, sunflower seeds, grated raw beetroot, 3 oz. (75g) cottage cheese, 1 jacket potato medium size
Mid-afternoon:	Soya savoury with carrots, cabbage, boiled beetroot (skinned when cooked)
Bedtime:	Red grape juice or 'Vecon'

N.B. When beetroot has been eaten in any quantity, stools and urine may appear pinkish red – quite normal, so do not be alarmed!

Menu 4 (days 7 and 8)

First thing: Lemon and honey drink or apple juice

Breakfast: Raw apple, fresh banana, yogurt –
                  amounts as suitable

Mid-morning: 1 teaspoonful of molasses in warm
                  water – or eaten off the spoon with
                  water to follow

Lunch: Salad as usual with *either* baked potato
                  or 1 slice wholewheat bread and
                  butter. 2 oz. (50g) milled nuts or 2-3
                  oz. (50-75g) cottage cheese and
                  chopped parsley

Mid-afternoon: China tea, or camomile herb tea,
                  apple or grape juice

Evening meal: Brown spaghetti with tomato sauce,
                  carrots, runner beans (in season) or
                  greens of some sort

Bedtime: 'Vecon' or red grape juice

Menu 5 (days 9 and 10)

First thing: Lemon and honey drink as before

Breakfast: Grated raw apple, tablespoonful
                  ground almonds, 2 tablespoonsful of
                  soaked raisins

Mid-morning: Molasses as before

Lunch: Salad as usual with either potato or
                  bread, and try 1-2 oz. (25-50g) grated
                  Cheddar or Cheshire cheese

Mid-afternoon: As usual

Evening meal: Herb almond pudding with carrots,
                  peas and green vegetable

Bedtime: 'Vecon' or red grape juice

Menu 6 (days 11 and 12)

First thing: Lemon and honey or juice of half fresh grapefruit
Breakfast: Bran flakes, fresh banana, dried milk
Mid-morning: Molasses and apple juice
Lunch: Salad with bread or potato and 1 hard boiled egg
Mid-afternoon: As usual – tea or fruit juice
Evening meal: Rice savoury, carrots, tomatoes, green vegetable
                  Sweet: yogurt and honey
Bedtime: 'Vecon' or grape juice.

N.B. Have bread or potato at lunch on alternate days, i.e. do not just keep to one type of starch because you happen to prefer it.

Menu 7 (days 13 and 14)

First thing: Apple juice
Breakfast: Half a grapefruit, 8-12 grapes, 1 apple, natural yogurt and honey
Mid-morning: 'Vecon' or molasses
Lunch: Salad with added dried raisins, 2-3 oz. (50-75g) Cheshire, Lancashire or Cheddar cheese
Mid-afternoon: As usual tea or fruit juice
Evening meal: Bean savoury, carrots, green vegetable.
                  Sweet: Baked apple and honey
Bedtime: 'Vecon' or grape juice

One month has now been completed, the patient will feel more secure, more energetic and will have gained one to four pounds in weight.

In the event of a recurrence of symptoms it would be advisable to return to the strict regime for a few days.

Maintenance Recipes

Brown (whole) Rice

> 3 tablespoonsful washed brown rice
> ½ pint (275ml) water
> ¼ teaspoonful of salt
> 1 teaspoonful of sunflower seed oil

Bring water, salt and oil to the boil, add washed rice and stir. Bring back to boil, cover and lower heat. Simmer 35-40 minutes or until water absorbed. This yields 6 tablespoonsful of cooked rice. (All tablespoons are level.)

Flavourings:
> Finely chopped mint
> Finely chopped parsley
> 'Vecon' or 'Barmene'
> Oregano
> Sage
> Honey
> Grated lemon rind

For the above
amount of rice:
> 1 teaspoonful of fresh herbs
> ½ teaspoonful of dried herbs
> 1 teaspoonful honey
> ½ teaspoonful lemon rind

Stewed Apple
Use Bramley cooking apples with a small amount of water to simmer, and honey to taste – but undersweeten in preference.

Apple Juice
It is better to use freshly made apple juice, but a good brand of bottled juice is all right, especially first thing in the morning. Remember to have fresh juice sometimes.

Soaked Raisins
Wash raisins well. Supermarket ones are soaked in mineral oil (liquid paraffin) to make them look glossy and weigh heavier. These need to be washed under running warm water and stirred around. When clean, put into a heat-proof bowl or basin, add a strip or two of lemon rind, then pour on boiling water just to cover them. Leave to soak overnight and they will be ready for the morning.

N.B. Always be sure to chew these raisins really well.

Salad Dressings
(1) 2 tablespoonsful sunflower seed oil
     1 tablespoonful of lemon juice
     1 teaspoonful of honey

Put all into a bottle, screw on lid, and shake

(2) 1 tablespoonful of oil
     1 tablespoonful of lemon juice
     2 tablespoonsful of natural yogurt
     1 teaspoonful of honey

Mix in same way.

Dried Bananas (from health food shops).
These will not need washing – so proceed as for raisins.

Savoury Millet (1-2 servings)
   1 clove garlic
   3 tomatoes
   1 level teaspoonful of 'Vecon' or 'Barmene'
   ½ pint (275ml) water
   1 teaspoonful of chopped, fresh parsley
   2 tablespoonsful of millet

Skin and slice tomatoes and put into a pan with water, crushed garlic and 'Vecon'. Bring to the boil, sprinkle in the millet and stir well. Cover and simmer for 10-15 minutes – liquor should be absorbed, but cook a few minutes longer if still 'soupy', stirring. Serve as soon as dry enough. Sprinkle on the fresh parsley and add the vegetables.

Soya and Barley Flakes (from health food shops).
Instructions for making porridge is on the packet. Generally: 1 cupful of flakes to 2 cupsful of water, simmer for 15-20 minutes. Make up milk from milk powder.

N.B. These flakes are useful in savouries and soups.

Soya Savoury
Prepared soya chunks or mince can be obtained at health food shops. Get the natural, unflavoured variety. Reconstitute the soya in liquor flavoured with 'Barmene' or 'Vecon', and crushed garlic. Follow instructions given, deleting onion at present – grated raw carrot added at

beginning of cooking helps to flavour, and also skinned
tomatoes (same as for millet).

Bean Savoury
Use adzuki beans – small brown beans. These should be
soaked either overnight or for 3-4 hours before using.
Pour off the soaking water. Add fresh made up
'Barmene' to cook:

    3 tablespoonsful of adzuki beans, soaked
    2 cloves crushed garlic
    2 skinned tomatoes
    ½ pint (275ml) 'Barmene'
    1 teaspoonful of honey
    1 tablespoonful of lemon juice

Simmer all together for 1 hour until the liquor is all
absorbed. Serve.

Rice Savoury
    2 tablespoonsful of brown rice
    1 teaspoonful of oil
    1 pint (500ml) boiling water and a little salt

Boil rice for 25 minutes, strain and rinse under hot
water. Return to pan, add:

    1 crushed clove garlic
    1 tablespoonful chopped fresh parsley
    ½ teaspoonful mixed herbs
    ½ grated apple
    1 tablespoonful of sunflower oil

Cover and shake pan while cooking for a further 15
minutes. Serve.

Herb Almond Pudding
   2 tablespoonsful of wholewheat breadcrumbs
   2 tablespoonsful of ground almonds
   1 teaspoonful of mixed herbs
   1 tablespoonful of chopped parsley
   1 egg
   1 cupful of made up 'Vecon' or 'Barmene'

Mix dry ingredients, beat egg in ½ cupful of liquor and add to dry ingredients. Beat well and use up rest of liquor to make a stiff batter. *Either* put into greased basin, cover and steam for 45 minutes *or* put into greased baking dish and bake at 375°F (191°C, Gas mark 4) for 25 minutes.

Brown Spaghetti (from health food shops).
Cook as instructed on packet.

Tomato Sauce
   3 skinned tomatoes
   1 clove crushed garlic
   1 teaspoonful of honey
   1 tablespoonful of oil
   ½ cupful of water

Cook all together for 10 minutes. If preferred thicker, add 2 teaspoonsful of brown rice flour sprinkled on and cook for 3-5 minutes more.

CHAPTER FIVE

PROGRESSIVE DIET

The diet can now assume normal lines. That is to say, of course, normal diet reform lines. The menus will be vegetarian, but meat, fish or poultry will be indicated in brackets for those feeling the need for flesh foods.

It is to be hoped that the improvement reached, so far, will be maintained without set-backs. There is no reason to expect them if one can maintain a relaxed unemotional and positive outlook, while enjoying life both at work and at home. There are bound to be problems and disagreements, but if these are coped with without suppressing them and 'bottling up' feelings, no reaction in the gut will occur; particularly now that the whole area has been renewed in healthy activity.

Where a choice is indicated on the menu, it is obviously better to vary your choice – the balance would be better with a variety. Though, to have two or three days on the same thing for economy's sake would be allowable.

Progressive Menus

Menu 1

First Thing: *Choice of:*
Lemon and honey
Bottled apple juice
Bottled water

Breakfast: ½ grapefruit
8-12 grapes
1 apple
Yogurt

Mid-morning: *Choice of:*
Tomato juice, grapefruit juice, 'Vecon', carrot juice, grape juice

Lunch: *Salad:*
Lettuce, water cress, pepper, tomato, grated carrot, grated beetroot, few raisins; 2 oz. (50g) milled nuts, sunflower seeds
One baked potato
Baked apple to follow

Mid-afternoon: China tea or herb tea

Evening Meal: Casserole of vegetables (grilled chop), carrots, cabbage and boiled rice
4-6 soaked prunes to follow

Bedtime: Grape juice, slippery elm or 'Vecon'

Menu 2

First Thing: *Choice of:*
Lemon and honey
Bottled apple juice
Bottled water

Breakfast:	1 boiled egg
	2 slices 100% wholewheat bread with butter (unsalted)
	1 apple
Mid-morning:	*Choice of:*
	'Vecon', grapefruit juice, carrot juice, grape juice
Lunch:	*Salad:*
	Lettuce, pepper, tomato, grated carrot, grated apple, sunflower seeds
	4 oz. (100g) cottage cheese
	1 slice 100% wholewheat bread with butter
	Soaked raisins and yogurt
Mid-afternoon:	China tea or herb tea
Evening Meal:	Cheese and onion savoury
	Broccoli
	Peas
	Soaked dried or fresh banana
Bedtime:	'Vecon', grape juice or slippery elm molasses and water

Menu 3

First Thing:	*Choice of:*
	Lemon and honey
	Bottled apple juice
	Bottled water
Breakfast:	Muesli with grated raw apple and yogurt
Mid-morning:	Coffee substitute, ½ milk, ½ water
Lunch:	*Salad:*
	Lettuce, cress, tomato, pepper, grated raw beetroot, celery
	2 oz. (50g) grated cheese

	1 potato, boiled or baked
	Molasses jelly and top of milk
Mid-afternoon:	China or herb tea
Evening Meal:	Moussaka with soya or beef mince
	Peas, cabbage, carrots
	Baked apple
Bedtime:	Grape juice or 'Vecon'
	Molasses and water

Menu 4

First Thing:	*Choice of:*
	Lemon and honey
	Bottled apple juice
	Bottled water
Breakfast:	Prunes and yogurt with ground almonds and honey
Mid-morning:	Coffee substitute or
	fruit juice or 'Vecon'
Lunch:	*Salad:*
	Celery, cooked beetroot, lettuce, dried pear, pepper, tomato
	Hard-boiled egg
	1 slice 100% wholewheat bread with butter
	1 homemade bun
Mid-afternoon:	China or herb tea or
	fruit juice
Evening Meal:	½ grapefruit
	Cheese, tomato and lentil rissoles (or grilled fish), chopped parsley, celery and carrots
	Baked apple
Bedtime:	Grape juice or coffee substitute
	Molasses and water

Menu 5

First Thing: *Choice of:*
                    Lemon and honey
                    Bottled apple juice
                    Bottled water

Breakfast: ½ grapefruit
                    1 pear
                    2 soaked dried bananas
                    Yogurt

Mid-morning: Coffee substitute
                    fruit juice or 'Vecon'

Lunch: *Salad:*
                    Lettuce or chinese leaves, tomato,
                    pepper, grated carrot, celery
                    4 oz. (100g) cottage cheese
                    Potato
                    Fresh apple

Mid-afternoon: China or herb tea or fruit juice

Evening Meal: ½ grapefruit
                    Cauliflower cheese
                    Tomatoes, carrots

Bedtime: Grape juice, 'Vecon' or coffee
                    substitute
                    Molasses and water

Menu 6

First Thing: *Choice of:*
                    Lemon and honey
                    Bottled apple juice
                    Bottled water

Breakfast: Prunes and yogurt
                    1-2 slices toast (100% wholewheat
                    bread), butter, honey

Mid-morning: Coffee substitute or 'Vecon',
                 Tomato juice
Lunch: *Salad:*
                 Lettuce, tomato, grated carrot, boiled
                 rice with chopped mint or chives,
                 peppers
                 2 oz. (50g) grated cheese
                 Homemade cake
Mid-afternoon: Tea or fruit juice
Evening Meal: Brown spaghetti with tomato sauce,
                 Cabbage, carrots
                 Fresh or baked apple
Bedtime: Grape juice or 'Vecon'
                 Molasses and water

Menu 7

First Thing: *Choice of:*
                 Lemon and honey
                 Bottled apple juice
                 Bottled water
Breakfast: ½ grapefruit
                 1 apple
                 1 peach or 8-12 grapes
                 Yogurt and honey
Mid-morning: Coffee substitute, 'Vecon' or fruit juice
Lunch: *Salad:*
                 Chinese leaves, pepper, cress, grated
                 carrot, few raisins, grated apple, 2 oz.
                 (50g) milled nuts, sunflower seeds
                 1 slice 100% wholewheat bread and
                 butter
                 Banana (fresh or dried)
Mid-afternoon: Tea or fruit juice

Evening Meal: Cheese and tomato quiche (chicken)
                   Peas, carrots, broccoli
                   Stewed or baked apple
Bedtime: Grape juice or 'Vecon'
                   Molasses and water

Menu 8

First Thing: Fruit juice
Breakfast: Bran flakes and milk with raisins
                   1 slice bread or toast
Mid-morning: Coffee substitute or tomato juice
Lunch: Good mixed salad with
                   hardboiled egg
                   Baked rice pudding
Mid-afternoon: Tea or fruit juice
Evening Meal: Vegetable and millet soup with grated
                   cheese
                   Compote of dried fruits and yogurt
Bedtime: Grape juice or 'Vecon'

Progressive Recipes

Baked Apple
Wash and core apple, score the skin twice, place in a tin
or oven proof dish in which there is just a covering of
water. Insert a teaspoonful of honey in the core hole.
Bake for 20-30 minutes at 400°F (204°C, gas mark 5)

Casserole of Vegetables (to serve 2)
    Ingredients:
    1 small onion
    1 tablespoonful of sunflower oil
    1 pepper, thinly chopped
    2 tomatoes, scalded and skinned

2 medium carrots, coarsely grated
2-3 sticks of celery, chopped
1 large courgette (or ⅓ cucumber), sliced
Clove garlic, crushed
¼ cabbage (shredded)
1 tablespoonful of sunflower seeds
1 mug made up 'Vecon' or 'Barmene'
(1 bare teaspoonful of Vecon dissolved in mug of hot water)

Turn on oven to 400°F (204°C, gas mark 5). First, cook the sliced onion and pepper in the sunflower oil, until onion looks transparent. Transfer to the casserole. Add the skinned tomatoes and all other ingredients. Pour over the liquor, cover and put into the oven. Cook for 30 minutes, then lower heat to 375° (194°C, gas mark 4) for another 45 minutes. Test to see if vegetables are tender. Sprinkle with a little grated cheese or ground almonds to serve.

Cheese and Onion Savoury (to serve 2)
Ingredients:
    1 small onion, sliced and chopped
    3 oz. (75g) grated cheddar cheese
    2 oz. (50g) soya flour
    2 oz. (50g) brown bread crumbs
    2 oz. (50g) brown rice flour
    1 egg
    2 tablespoonsful sunflower oil
    ½ teaspoonful of salt
    ½ teaspoonful of dried sage or 1 teaspoonful of fresh, chopped

Mix the flours and breadcrumbs, add salt and herbs, add onion and cheese then the oil and egg beaten together. The mixture should be a stiff dropping consistency, i.e. just dropping off the fork – but not easily. Put the mixture into a greased basin – tie down with greaseproof paper, then metal foil (or a cloth) and steam in boiling water (halfway up basin) for 1 hour.

Muesli
There is a fashion at present to use the various brands of muesli from the packet with added milk and fruit. This can be difficult to digest. The original Bircher Muesli stipulated that the oat flakes (wheat or barley or soya, as the case may be) should be soaked overnight – *then* the chopped nuts, raisins, grated raw apple and skimmed milk added with a little muscavado sugar (dark brown or unrefined sugar).

Molasses Jelly
    ½ pint (275ml) water
    2 tablespoonsful of molasses (or black treacle)
    1 rounded teaspoonful of agar-agar

Bring water to boil and dissolve molasses in it. Sprinkle in the agar and stir simmering 2-3 minutes. Remove from heat and divide into small dishes.

N.B. A little grated lemon rind can be added to the cold water before boiling, to give extra flavour.

Moussaka (Serves 2)
Ingredients:
   4 oz. (100g) soya natural mince (or 6 oz. (175g) beef
   mince, pre-cooked)
   (reconstituted in a cup of made up 'Barmene'
   plus 1 crushed clove of garlic and ¼ teaspoonful of salt)
   4 oz. (100g) mushrooms, sliced
   2 tomatoes scalded and skinned and sliced
   3-4 medium potatoes, scrubbed well
   1 teaspoonful of thyme
   1 tablespoonful of sunflower oil

Grease appropriate-sized oven dish or tin. Thinly slice a
potato and line the dish. Pour in half the mince, add a
layer of mushrooms and tomatoes and a sprinkling of
thyme – another layer of thinly sliced potato – the rest of
the mince with mushrooms and tomato and thyme.
Finish with topping of potato and the oil. Bake in
moderate oven 375°, gas mark 4 for 35-45 minutes.

Fruit Buns or Cake
Ingredients:
   2 oz. (50g) soya flour
   2 oz. (50g) rice flour
   2 oz. (50g) ground almonds
   2 oz. (50g) 100% wholewheat flour
   4 oz. (100g) margarine
   4 tablespoonsful sunflower oil
   3 eggs
   4 oz. (100g) muscavado sugar
   or 2 oz. (50g) honey and 2 oz. (50g) sugar
   3-4 oz. (75-100g) fruit – currants, sultanas, raisins
   1 lemon, grated rind and juice

Mix together all flours and the almonds. In another bowl cream the fats together then add the sugar/honey and cream well. Add one egg at a time, plus 1 tablespoonful of flour and beat well to a light and foaming consistency. Now fold in the remaining flour, the fruit and lemon rind and juice and put into prepared bun tins or a cake tin and *either* (for buns) bake at 400°F (204°C, gas mark 5) for 15-20 minutes *or* (for cake) bake at 375°F (191°C, gas mark 4) for 1-hour.

Alternative flavouring – use black treacle as sweetener, with 1 teaspoonful mixed spice instead of lemon.

Cheese, Tomato and Lentil Rissoles
Ingredients:
- 4 oz. (100g) red lentils, well soaked (3-4 hours)
- 3 oz. (75g) grated cheddar cheese
- 3 tomatoes, scalded and skinned
- 1 teaspoonful tomato purée
- 1 teaspoonful of muscavado sugar
- ½ teaspoonful of salt
- 1-2 cloves garlic, crushed (according to taste)
- 1 egg
- ¼ teaspoonful of oregano
- Bran, sunflower oil

Simmer lentils until soft, then leave to cool. Add cheese, tomatoes, purée, sugar and salt, garlic and oregano. Mix well together, add beaten egg to bind. Shape into rissoles, dip into bran and dry 'fry' or grill fairly slowly for 7 minutes each side. Add small amount of sunflower oil to baste and prevent from sticking. Sprinkle with chopped parsley and serve.

Cauliflower Cheese (Serves 4)
Break up cauliflower into florets and par-boil 5 minutes in slightly salted water. Remove and drain and pile into oven dish with sauce and bake 15-20 minutes at 375°F (191°C, gas mark 4).

Sauce:
    ½ pint (275ml) milk
    Pat of butter
    1 tablespoonful of brown rice flour
    3 oz. (75g) of cheddar cheese, grated
    Breadcrumbs or bran to top

Heat milk and butter, stir in rice flour. Bring to boil and cook 3 minutes. Remove from heat and mix in cheese. Pour over cauliflower, sprinkle over crumbs or bran and bake.

Cheese and Tomato Quiche
Pastry is used in this recipe – but if it appears on the menu only once in a week it should be tolerated. Made with these wholesome ingredients it makes less demands on the digestion.

Ingredients:
    2 oz. (50g) 100% wholewheat flour
    2 oz. (50g) rice flour 100%
    1 oz. (25g) cheddar cheese grated
    2-3 tablespoonsful of sunflower oil
    Water to mix

Mix the flours in a bowl. Add the grated cheese. Mix in the oil with a knife and then with a wire pastry blender.

Add water to mix to a stiff dough. Prepare small flan tin. Collect dough into a ball and put onto floured board. 'Knuckle' it down to required size and thickness to line flan tin (this is better than rolling).

Filling:
    3-4 tomatoes according to size
    3 oz. (75g) cheddar cheese, grated
    2 eggs
    ½ pint milk
    Clove garlic

Scald and skin tomatoes. Slice into the flan and cover with cheese. Beat eggs in milk with crushed garlic. Pour over tomatoes and cheese – but not to overflow!

Bake in fairly hot oven at 425°F (218°C, gas mark 6) for 20 minutes. Lower heat to 400°F (204°C, gas mark 5) for 10-15 minutes. If not quite set allow another 5 minutes with lower heat still.

Baked Rice Pudding
Ingredients:
    3 level tablespoonsful of brown rice (well washed)
    1 pint (550ml) milk
    2 tablespoonsful (level) of honey or dark sugar

The dark sugar tends to curdle the milk so this pudding needs to be cooked very slowly.

Blend all ingredients together and bake at 300°F (149°C, gas mark 1-2) for 2½ hours.